Allen Carr

No more
diets

Allen Carr

No more diets

ARCTURUS

ARCTURUS

This edition published in 2017 by Arcturus Publishing Limited
26/27 Bickels Yard, 151–153 Bermondsey Street,
London SE1 3HA, UK

ISBN: 978-1-84837-554-3
AD000038UK

Printed in the UK

To Cris Hay whose contribution to this book was invaluable

ALLEN CARR

In 1983 Allen Carr was a successful businessman and entrepreneur, enjoying a lifestyle that most people would envy. An accountant by training and profession, he was one of life's achievers. In one respect, however, he was an abject failure: he could not stop smoking. Indeed after each of his countless failed attempts, he smoked more and ended up smoking 100 cigarettes a day. Then the inescapable logic of Easyway took root in his brain, and Allen's life took another dramatic turn.

Convinced that his method could help others as effectively as it had helped him, Allen set about turning Easyway into a universal program for helping smokers kick their addiction. If he, a heavy smoker for over 30 years, could stop easily and painlessly, then other smokers could as well. Now, many years later, Easyway is recognized around the world as the brand leader in stopping smoking therapies. Allen soon realized that his method could be applied to many other kinds of addictions, difficulties and fears.

His own attempts at weight loss had, for various reasons, been unsuccessful and he originally thought the Easyway method could not be applied to weight loss. However, the simple nature of the method – that with the correct frame of mind any behaviour can be changed – made him realize how it could and Easyweigh was born.

INTRODUCTION

In 1983 I discovered something every smoker dreams of: an easy way to stop smoking. I quit my previous career, and set out to cure the world of smoking. I am now widely regarded as the world's leading expert on helping smokers quit. My book, *The Easy Way to Stop Smoking,* has sold over ten million copies, and my network of clinics spans the globe.

But my success has not been limited to smokers. I soon realized my method was equally effective for any kind of drug addiction. In fact, I was delighted to discover that the method could be applied to almost any kind of problem.

Before I discovered the information contained in this book, most of my attempts to lose weight were short-lived. While weight loss was my main objective, everything was fine. But whenever I was faced with some seemingly more urgent project, my resolution weakened. I would return to the same eating habits, and hence the same weight, as before. Consequently for many years I believed that being overweight was the one problem that could not be solved by my method. The essence of the method is that with the correct frame of mind it's very easy to get completely free of any kind of addictive behaviour, once and for all. But you can't stop eating.

Fortunately, you don't have to. What happened to make me realize my method would work for weight control? I owe it all to a squirrel.

THE SQUIRREL

He climbed the garden wall to escape from my cat. The next week I saw him tucking into the peanuts meant for the birds. I thought, 'Eat too many of those, my friend, and next time you won't be able to climb the wall.' But to my surprise he suddenly stopped eating the nuts and started storing them.

How did he know when to stop eating?

WILD ANIMALS

Picture in your mind a school of fish, a herd of gazelles, or a pride of lions. The animals might well be of different sizes, but within their species they are always the same shape. You might see skinny ones when food is short, but you never see obese ones when food is in abundance. Obesity is a problem for only two categories of being: the most intelligent species on the planet, and the animals we domesticate.

MY CLAIM

You can eat as much of your favourite foods as you want to, as often as you want to, and be the exact weight that you want to be. You can achieve this without having to diet or undertake a special exercise regime, without using willpower or gimmicks, and without feeling deprived and miserable.

YOU WILL ONLY ACHIEVE MY CLAIM IF YOU FOLLOW ALL THE INSTRUCTIONS

The first instruction is to open your mind. From birth we are brainwashed to hold certain beliefs about eating and food. My method, which I call 'Easyweigh', is based on common sense. You won't need expert knowledge about calories or vitamins.

Perhaps you feel my claim is extravagant. But that's what over 99.99 per cent of creatures on this planet achieve. Providing their favourite foods are available, they eat as much as they want whenever they want, and are never overweight.

WHERE DID I GO WRONG?

I failed to make the distinction between eating and overeating. Eating is vital for survival. It's a genuinely pleasant pastime that can and should be enjoyed throughout our lives. Overeating is a serious, self-inflicted disease that shortens life and ruins its quality. It destroys self-respect and spoils the great pleasure of eating.

THE SUBTLETY OF THE TRAP

The problem creeps up on us so gradually that we barely notice it happening. Imagine going to bed healthy and energetic, with not an ounce of fat on your body, and waking up pot-bellied, bloated and lethargic. You'd rush to your doctor in horror, wondering what awful disease you had suddenly developed.

See obesity that way – as a terrible, life-threatening disease! Don't be fooled by the fact that it took years to progress this far, and don't make the fatal mistake of assuming that one day soon you'll get round to doing something about it.

HOW CAN MY CLAIM POSSIBLY BE TRUE?

Perhaps you're thinking, 'But I already eat as much of my favourite foods as I want! That's why I'm overweight! So how can Easyweigh change the situation?"

Remember I asked you to open your mind. Read the claim again. It's not a bad package. If doubt should creep in, remind yourself that 99.99 per cent of creatures achieve it. Do you rate your intelligence below theirs?

DIETS DON'T WORK

They just turn what should be a very pleasant activity into an absolute nightmare. The only thing you can think about between meals is food, and when lunchtime finally arrives you're depressed because you can't eat the quantity or type of food that you would like. You're miserable every time you stray from your diet, and only slightly less miserable when you stick to it. Even if you do somehow stick to it for long enough to lose the excess weight, the chances are you soon return to your previous eating habits, and the weight piles back on depressingly quickly – far faster than it came off!

HAVE YOU A FEELING OF FOREBODING?

Then dismiss it straightaway. Easyweigh is not a diet. The object is not merely to lose weight, but to enjoy life! Once you're bursting with energy, feel proud of your figure and enjoy every meal, then life will become the pleasure that it's meant to be. You aren't going to go hungry – far from it – so there's no need to feel deprived and miserable. You're about to start a whole new wonderful life!

'HOW LONG DOES EASYWEIGH TAKE?'

One of the beauties of Easyweigh is that you don't have to wait to achieve your object before you get excited. You solved your weight problem the moment you started reading this book. All you have to do is follow the instructions. The first was to open your mind. The second is to start off, right now, with a feeling of excitement.

MOTHER NATURE'S *GOOD FOOD GUIDE*

I have referred to the problem as overeating. This might suggest that you won't be allowed to eat as much as you want. Not so. There are two common misconceptions about eating. We'll deal with the second later. The first is that obesity is caused by eating too much. In fact, the real cause is eating foods that don't contain enough nutrients and energy, and therefore leave you hungry, even when you feel full. This makes you keep eating.

All creatures instinctively know how to survive, and knowing which foods to eat is an essential part of that. Each species has its own specialized digestive system. One species' food is another species' poison.

THE INCREDIBLE MACHINE

The human body is the most sophisticated survival machine on the planet. It's the result of three billion years of trial and error.

For all our advanced technology humans cannot create a single living cell, let alone trillions of cells working in harmony.

If the total duration of life on earth were represented by a single year, we wouldn't have known that vitamins and calories even existed until the last fraction of the last second on the last day. How did we survive for so long without nutritionists?

Funnily enough, it's only within that minuscule fraction of human history that obesity has become the epidemic that it now is.

THE SO-CALLED EXPERTS

Once we are weaned, other members of
the supposedly intelligent human race tell us
what to eat. Their opinions are affected by
massive commercial interests, prejudice and
ignorance. When health professionals give
advice that contradicts three billion years of
trial and error, they can hardly be described
as intelligent!

I'm not denying the human race's
extraordinary ingenuity in curing disease. I'm
just saying that prevention is better than cure:
perhaps pride in our progress has blinded
us to the fact that many diseases are self-
inflicted. There are just three causes of death
among wild animals: violent death, disease
and old age. By contrast many humans seem
all too ready to dig themselves into an early
grave with their knife and fork.

HOW DO ANIMALS KNOW WHAT TO EAT?

Imagine you are Mother Nature. You've blessed the planet with a myriad of wonderful species. How would you ensure that they know the difference between food and poison?

A clever way would be to make food taste good and poison taste foul. And that, of course, is exactly what she did.

'WHAT ABOUT ACQUIRED TASTES?'

Like coffee and beer? Beware of them! They prove my point. Wild animals wouldn't touch them. Supposedly intelligent human beings persevere, and become dependent on caffeine and alcohol.

Most teenagers find they cannot acquire the taste for coffee without liberal doses of sugar to help it down. They might well cut out the sugar later, but if coffee really tasted good they wouldn't need to add it in the first place. And to say you enjoy the taste of a pint of bitter is a contradiction in terms. My dictionary defines bitter as a 'sharp and unpleasant taste'.

THE OTHER SENSES

Mother Nature has also equipped us with sight, smell and touch. Along with taste they help us to decide whether something is food or poison. If it looks good, smells good and tastes good, it's food. A pet cat will first peer at its food, then sniff it, then taste a morsel. Depending upon the conclusion it has reached it will either tuck in or walk away in disdain as if you've fed it poison.

The system is so ingenious, that when good food goes off, we get a warning sign. When fruit rots, it looks, smells, tastes and feels awful. You could be deceived by the look and feel of a bad egg, so Nature increases the bad smell to prevent you from eating poison.

WHY DO WE NEED TO EAT?

That's obvious: we'd die if we didn't. But we need to delve deeper. The reasons are twofold. We need food to replace the millions of our cells that die each day, and to provide the energy to carry out our daily life. Just as a car needs fuel and maintenance to transport you from A to B, so your body needs them to transport you through life.

WHY DO OTHER SPECIES EAT?

After all, they don't know that you have to eat to survive. All mothers know the difficulty of trying to persuade a baby or child to eat if it doesn't want to. I've explained how each species knows which foods to eat, but how does Mother Nature ensure they have a desire to eat in the first place?

The answer, of course, is that she equipped them with an ingenious device called hunger!

ONE OF NATURE'S INGENIOUS DEVICES

We tend to think of hunger as an evil. Start seeing it for what it is: a friend for life! We are led to believe that there is pleasure in eating for eating's sake, or because food just tastes good, regardless of whether or not we are hungry. But in fact the only real pleasure in eating is in ending your hunger. That's why the French say, '*Bon appetit!*' when you sit down to one of their lovingly prepared meals. They know that if you don't bring a 'good appetite' to the table, all their hard work will have been wasted: you just won't enjoy the food.

TRY EATING PORTION AFTER PORTION OF YOUR FAVOURITE FOOD

Eat enough and you'll soon get sick of it – perhaps even literally. But if you're starving, even a rat becomes a delicacy.

While we're on the subject of starvation, let's dispose of a common red herring. We've all met people who blame their problem on their glands or their metabolism. You know the sort of thing: 'I don't eat enough to feed a sparrow but the pounds keep piling on.' Try telling that to Bob Geldof! Just one glance at the news footage that moved him to 'feed the world' proves such statements to be utterly phoney.

Starving people are never overweight, regardless of their glands, metabolism or genetic disposition. There is only one cause of obesity: eating the wrong foods!

THE SOPHISTICATION OF HUNGER

Hunger is not just a matter of our bodies telling us we need to eat. Wild animals crave different types of food depending on which nutrients are deficient in their diets. The 'fancies' that pregnant women experience are the result of their bodies demanding additional nutrients to feed their developing babies.

THE BEAUTY OF HUNGER

Between meals your body's supply of energy and nutrients gradually runs down. Providing you satisfy your hunger with the right foods, then most of the time you won't even be aware of this process. When you do become aware of feeling hungry, you can relish the genuine pleasure of satisfying that hunger. You can enjoy this marvellous pleasure a number of times every single day for the rest of your life, together with an abundance of energy and health, without ever being overweight.

But you will only reap all these marvellous benefits if you eat correctly.

WILD ANIMALS ONLY EAT WHEN THEY ARE HUNGRY

They stop eating when they have satisfied their hunger.

Compare this behaviour to that of humans. Once we're weaned, our eating behaviour is dictated by our parents. 'You'll not leave the table until you've cleared your plate.' At this impressionable age we are already being ordered to overeat. Our eating habits are further moulded by the school we attend, the job we take, the partner we choose … and so on.

WHAT WEIGHT DO YOU WANT TO BE?

That's easy: it's the weight you happen to be when you can admire your naked reflection in a mirror.

When you see someone in their swimwear, do you need to know their weight to know whether they are overweight?

If you have a preconceived weight, you're following humans' guide, not Mother Nature's. Wild animals don't have scales – at least not the kind for weighing yourself!

'SHOULD I THROW AWAY MY SCALES?'

No! The most sinister aspect of the trap is that weight gain is so gradual as to be imperceptible day by day. The same is true of weight *loss*: we appear no slimmer than the day before. This can be disheartening, so record your weight now, and get someone to take your photograph in a swimming costume. Weigh yourself regularly: I suggest once a week, and at roughly the same time each week. Record your progress. Seeing it written down in black and white will prove that Easyweigh is working, and encourage you to keep applying its principles.

THE SECOND OF THE TWO COMMON MISCONCEPTIONS

The first was that obesity is caused by overeating, when in fact it's caused by *incorrect* eating: the consumption of junk foods that don't contain enough nutrients and energy, and therefore leave you unsatisfied, reaching for more.

The second misconception is that the foods that are bad for you are the ones that taste best.

I have very good news for you: underneath all the brainwashing and conditioning, the healthiest, most nutritious foods are also the foods that taste the most delicious. Remember that wild animals eat the foods that taste the best to *them*, and they are never overweight!

WHAT ARE YOUR FAVOURITE FOODS?

Look back on your life and ask yourself if your tastes have changed over time. We acquire a taste for whichever foods we eat regularly. That's why mother's cooking always tastes the best.

Do you think it's coincidence that most Asians just happen to like rice, that most Italians enjoy pasta, that most Brits tend to favour bread and potatoes?

Do you realize that if you had been brought up in another country you would have a very different set of favourite foods?

FREE YOURSELF FROM SLAVERY TO YOUR TASTE BUDS

If you mistakenly give someone who's cut it out just a few grains of sugar in their tea, they'll grimace as if you'd laced it with arsenic.

The beautiful truth is that our taste buds are flexible. Just as youngsters persevere to 'acquire' a taste for poisons like tobacco and alcohol, so we've been brainwashed to believe that junk foods taste good. But fortunately it works both ways. You can also acquire a taste for the foods that will keep you slim and healthy for the rest of your life.

DO YOU FEEL CHEATED?

I've asked you not to have a preconceived target weight. I'm also going to ask you to drop your preconceptions about what will become your favourite foods.

Perhaps you feel I've moved the goal-posts. I claimed you could eat as much of your favourite foods as often as you want to, and be the exact weight you want to be.

YOU CAN DO EXACTLY THAT!

Remember that I also asked to open your mind.

This is the most challenging thing I will ask you to do: to reverse the lifetime's brainwashing. From birth we all receive a mass of information about food and eating habits, and much of it is false. Sometimes the brainwashing is passed on inadvertently by people who have our best interests at heart, for example, our parents or health professionals. Sometimes the brainwashing is deliberately exploited for profit, by the hugely powerful conglomerates in the food industry.

YOU NEED TO USE YOUR INTELLIGENCE AND YOUR IMAGINATION

The rewards are wonderful. Genuine food will taste better. The pleasure of eating will be greatly enhanced once you know you're consuming food that keeps you fit and healthy – food that satisfies your hunger without causing obesity and all the other diseases associated with incorrect eating. You'll enjoy every meal with a clear conscience.

DO YOU TREAT YOUR BODY LIKE A ROLLS ROYCE OR A WASTE-DISPOSAL UNIT?

Would you dream of filling the petrol tank of your car with diesel, or topping up the engine with dirty oil? Of course not! If you did, the vehicle wouldn't last very long. Yet we treat our most precious possession – the vehicle upon which the length and quality of our life depends – like a waste-disposal unit. We shove all sorts of junk down one end, blindly trusting that it will come out the other.

'BUT I'VE SURVIVED SO FAR!'

True – but it's no thanks to you. It's because your body is such an incredible machine. You can actually swallow harmful substances, provided they're not too harmful, and your body will cope. But it wouldn't be able to cope if you did it every day! Don't forget that you're reading this book because your body is having a hard time coping.

If you could get a glimpse inside your body to see the problems you create for it when you eat incorrectly, you wouldn't even need to finish the book – you'd stop doing it straightaway.

THE DIGESTIVE SYSTEM

The purpose of the digestive system is to extract the energy and nutrients from food, and dispose of the waste materials using a minimum of energy.

One of the many incredible things about living creatures is that the process of digestion is carried out subconsciously and simultaneously with many other survival functions. Digestion uses more energy than any other single function. This is why we feel sleepy after a large meal. Some foods, such as meat, require more energy to digest than they give in return.

THE 'PLASTIC BUCKET' SYNDROME

Most cars run on a mixture of petrol, vapour and air. Petrol is refined from crude oil. So is plastic. But if you ran out of petrol, would you cut up a plastic bucket, shove the pieces into the petrol tank, and expect the engine to start?

That's effectively what we do when we eat junk food.

'FOR STRONG TEETH AND BONES DRINK MILK'

A typical 'plastic bucket' myth.

We need calcium for strong teeth and bones. Milk and dairy products contain calcium. But how do cows obtain their calcium? Elephants have the largest teeth, in the form of tusks, and also the largest bones. But adult elephants don't drink milk nor do adult cows.

Apart from the pets we domesticate, we are the only species that drinks the milk of other creatures.

'FOR BIG, TOUGH MUSCLES EAT STEAK'

We need protein to survive, so we eat cows.
It sounds logical, but the digestive system
just doesn't work that way. Where do the
cows get their protein from? The largest,
strongest animals on the planet – such as
elephants, hippos and horses – do not eat
meat. The body produces the protein it
needs from the food consumed.

We also need iron. But would you dream of
eating iron filings?

'DOES THIS MEAN WE MUST EAT GRASS?'

No! A cow eats grass because its digestive system is designed to extract the nutrients it needs from that particular food source. Mother Nature has provided each species with a specialized food package which supplies it with the nutrients and energy it needs and a specialized digestive system to match.

Humans are just another species. Like all other species, you'll eat your favourite foods, provided they are available.

WHAT IS JUNK FOOD?

Forget about the usual definition of junk food, and of how a doctor or nutritionist might define it. For the purposes of Easyweigh, junk food is any food that isn't part of the food package specifically designed for our particular species.

But how do we know what is in that package? How can we know what is real food for humans, and what is junk?

Fortunately there is irrefutable evidence to guide us. Let's start reversing the brainwashing.

'DOES YOUR FAMILY GET ENOUGH MEAT IN THEIR DIET?'

When I was a lad, mothers had the fear of God put into them with this question. Back then, red meat, butter and double cream were considered health foods. Nowadays most experts regard these foods as a recipe for disaster. But they can't completely escape the meat-and-dairy mind-set: rather than endorse an entirely different set of foods, they recommend lean cuts of meat, chicken, and low-fat dairy products. I find that suspect. It's like saying: 'Cut down on the arsenic,' or, 'Switch to strychnine because it's less poisonous.'

We have already exploded the myth that you need to eat meat in order to obtain protein. The largest, strongest and most energetic land animals are all herbivores.

'BUT WHO IS KING OF THE JUNGLE?'

A lion is nowhere nearly as strong as an elephant, and in case your idea of a lion is a creature bursting with energy, bear in mind that it sleeps for 20 hours a day. An orangutan, which does not eat meat, sleeps for only six. Besides, any energy the lion does possess, it didn't obtain from eating meat.

CARNIVORES DON'T EAT CARNIVORES

Lions kill leopards and cheetahs but don't usually eat them. Upon making a kill the first thing the dominant member of the pride does is rip open its victim's stomach and eat its contents. That's where a lion gets most of its protein from – the vegetation eaten by herbivores. After the contents of the stomach, the lion opts for juicy organs such as the heart, liver, kidneys, intestines and brains. Flesh is the last choice. It's usually creatures at the bottom of the pecking order, such as hyenas and vultures, that are left with the flesh.

LOOK AT THE FACTS

Bear in mind that cooking is a relatively
recent innovation in human development.
Try eating raw meat! Carnivores have fangs,
molars that slice rather than grind, and
long sharp claws designed to tear raw flesh.
Human beings don't possess these so they
can only eat meat if they cook it and even
then they find it hard to digest.

Carnivores produce ten times more acid in
their stomachs than humans. The acid breaks
down the meat and the toxins it contains.

Meat putrefies quickly, so carnivores have
relatively short intestines to dispose of the
decomposing meat in the shortest possible
time. We have over 30 feet of intestines.

WE AREN'T EVEN EMOTIONALLY EQUIPPED TO EAT MEAT

We have neither the stomach to eat animals, nor the wish to kill them. Most meat-eaters agree that if they were asked to kill a farm animal they couldn't do it. This, of course, is why we have to try and fool ourselves with the language we use. We don't eat 'cow', 'hen', 'deer', 'calf' or 'pig'. We eat 'beef', 'chicken', 'venison', 'veal' and 'pork'.

I'M NOT TRYING TO APPEAL TO YOUR CONSCIENCE

And I'm not saying you have to become vegetarian. I'm saying that as far as human beings are concerned, meat is junk. But there are no restrictions with Easyweigh. It's based on natural principles, and sometimes wild animals have to eat junk when their favourite foods are scarce. Because they eat real food most of the time, they are never overweight. The beauty of Easyweigh is that there is what I call a 'junk margin' – which means that as long as 70% of what you eat is real food, the remainder can be junk without doing much harm.

I'm appealing to your common sense to help you see that we are not natural carnivores.

GIVE A CHILD AN APPLE AND A SPARROW

If it eats the bird and plays with the apple I'll eat my hat! But which would your pet cat eat?

When you see a newborn lamb in the spring, are you overcome with some primitive urge to tear its throat out and gorge on the blood and gore? Or do you turn to your companion and say: 'Ah! Just look at that!'

WE LOVE ANIMALS

We would rather starve ourselves than see our pets starve. But at the same time we are breeding animals that trust us purely so we can slaughter and eat them!

It wouldn't be so bad if there weren't ample supplies of genuine food. Furthermore, meat makes us overweight, unhealthy and lethargic.

MEAT HAS VERY LITTLE GOING FOR IT

It provides very little energy. Energy comes from carbohydrates: meat has virtually none. It also contains very little fibre. Fibre is essential to good digestion and health. Meat is the most difficult food to digest, and the body has to work particularly hard to dispose of its wastes.

But what about the marvellous taste?

Well, if cooked meat tastes so gorgeous, why do we feel the need to season it? Why the need for mint, apple or cranberry sauce? Why do we often add overpoweringly strong flavours such as horseradish, mustard, spices and garlic to meat?

It's either to add flavour to an otherwise bland taste or to disguise a foul taste.

'BUT VEGETARIANS ALWAYS LOOK SO PASTY AND UNHEALTHY!'

If that is indeed true it's not because they don't eat meat. It's because some vegetarians, having forsaken meat, feel that gives them *carte blanche* to eat absolutely anything else instead. Many people become vegetarian as students, and having done so they adopt a diet of crisps and chocolate and very little else! In fact, many converts to vegetarianism replace the meat in their diet with large amounts of cheese and dairy products.

'DRINKA PINTA MILKA DAY!'

Not so long ago all schoolchildren were
provided with a third of a pint of milk
each day – even though some pupils were
obviously allergic to it.

I found it quite a challenge to reverse my
own brainwashing, and accept that meat
was junk. With milk and dairy products, the
challenge was even greater.

For the first few months of our lives we drink
only milk. How can milk and dairy products
possibly be junk?

THE FIRST IRREFUTABLE FACT

Although all baby mammals thrive on their mothers' milk, it's part of Nature's plan that they be weaned. The enzymes necessary to break down and digest milk are rennin and lactase. They are all but gone by the age of three in most humans. Our bodies aren't designed to digest milk once we have been weaned.

Can you think of any adult animals, apart from human beings and domesticated pets, that drink milk?

THE SECOND IRREFUTABLE FACT

Milk is not just one substance: that of each species is different. The milk of one is unsuitable for another.

Cow's milk is a natural food, but only for calves. Would you drink it warm straight from the udder?

All milk contains casein, which coagulates in the stomach to form large, tough, dense curds which are difficult to digest. Cows' milk has 300 times more casein than human milk. You impose an enormous burden on your digestive and waste-disposal systems if you drink milk.

NATURAL FOOD VERSUS JUNK

Now we've established that meat and dairy products are junk, it doesn't take Sherlock Holmes to deduce that what's left is fruit, vegetables, nuts, seeds, wheat, rice and other grains. Strictly speaking, even grains are junk because they're not normally eaten in their natural state, but have to be cooked. Real or 'natural' foods are those that can easily be eaten and digested raw, in their entirely natural state. Junk foods are those that have to be processed in some way.

Natural foods are the way Mother Nature intended; junk foods have been interfered with by humans.

PERHAPS YOU FIND ALL THIS RATHER DAUNTING

If so, remind yourself of the claim and the junk margin. I'm not saying you can only eat raw, natural foods. I'm merely saying that fruit, vegetables, nuts and seeds are the *ideal* foods for human consumption. Please also bear in mind that there is a spectrum within the junk margin: technically wholemeal bread is junk because it has been processed, but it's a far higher grade of junk than chocolate, for example.

We have devised numerous methods of processing food. You can cook it, refine it, freeze it, smoke it, can it, pickle it, bottle it, season it, sweeten it, dry it, or saturate it with salt or other additives.

WE PROCESS FOODS FOR VARIOUS REASONS

Sometimes it's to help us digest certain foods, such as meat, which would otherwise be inedible. Sometimes it's to extract poisonous contents. The main reason is to prevent it from decomposing.

In other words, the chief object of processing food is to render it inedible to bacteria. But if it's not good enough for bacteria, then it's probably not good enough for you and me!

BEWARE OF PROCESSED FOODS

If your car's handbook specified a certain grade of petrol you would follow the advice. Every time we process natural food we ignore the advice of an intelligence a billion times greater than our own.

One of the unfortunate side effects of processing natural food is that it tends to destroy the food's valuable high water content.

THE VITAL WATER CONTENT

The fuel and lubricants of a car are liquids.
Liquidity plays an equally important role in
the smooth running of your body. Blood
transports energy and essential chemicals
to the whole of your body. Liquidity is
also extremely important for digestion and
disposal of waste.

By far the most common means of
processing food is to cook it. Unfortunately,
cooking tends to kill the nutrients in the
food and reduce the water content. Drinking
during the meal or adding water while
cooking unfortunately does not negate the
effect. That's 'plastic bucket' thinking. Your
digestive system just doesn't work that way.

THE ONE VALID REASON TO PROCESS FOOD

Since all processing of natural food detracts from its nutritional value, the only valid reason to preserve food is to provide against famine. Pioneer sailors survived on cheese, biscuits, jam and salted meat. But they soon learned that if they were deprived of fresh fruit and vegetables for long periods, serious disease was the result.

Much of our food is processed by giant commercial conglomerates. Reflect on what you've eaten in the past week. What percentage was natural food? Even staples like milk, bread and potatoes have been processed. Wild animals only eat junk when the real McCoy isn't available. No wonder so many of us are obese, lethargic and unhealthy.

THE EFFECTS OF EATING TOO MUCH JUNK

You become bloated, but because you've failed to provide the energy and nutrients your body needs, you're still hungry. So you consume more junk and feel even worse. Junk food provides little energy while using up a lot, because the body has to work so hard to digest it and dispose of the waste. Your kidneys and liver can't remove all the toxins and your stomach, intestines, and bowels cannot cope with the permanent overload. The ever-increasing toxic surplus has to be stored in your body as fat. You become permanently tired and unhealthy, and ironically, permanently hungry.

So what's the answer? What are ideal foods for humans?

WHAT DO OUR CLOSEST RELATIONS EAT?

Our DNA is over 99% identical to that of a chimpanzee. We are remarkably similar in appearance to our cousins, the great apes, and our digestive organs are virtually the same.

Doesn't the fact that we possess virtually identical digestive systems suggest that we should eat the same foods?

If they can get them, gorillas like to eat fresh fruit and nuts. If they can't get fresh fruit, they will supplement their diet with other vegetation. They never eat meat or dairy products. Some apes very occasionally eat meat but the vast bulk of their diet consists of fruit, nuts and other vegetation.

'HOW COULD YOU SURVIVE ON JUST FRUIT?'

Our so-called need for dense food is just part of the brainwashing. All baby mammals develop at a prodigious rate on nothing but their mother's milk. And if you're concerned about vitamin deficiency, let me reassure you that one of the beauties of Easyweigh is that you don't have to worry about vitamins or fat grams or counting calories.

An adult male gorilla is 30 times stronger than a man. How did the human race manage to survive before it discovered fire and vitamins? Use your common sense.

ALL THE EVIDENCE POINTS TO FRUIT

That's what our ancestors ate, and that's what our nearest cousins eat today. That was our staple diet before we left the forests and cleared them to farm crops and livestock. That's what our babies are weaned on even today. Children naturally love fruit, and so would adults if they hadn't been brainwashed.

THE PROOF IS IN THE PUDDING

Fruit genuinely tastes good. That's why we use it to flavour so many other foods. We add fruit flavours to many meat dishes: duck a l'orange, ham and pineapple, turkey with redcurrant jelly, pork with apple sauce. We use it to flavour alcoholic drinks, to sweeten the pill. Those jellies and ice creams we loved as kids were usually fruit-flavoured. We crown cheesecakes and pastries and other 'delicacies' with fresh fruit. And what are the most popular flavours for milkshakes? Banana, strawberry, pineapple, etc.

WHY NOT EAT THE REAL McCOY?

Why eat a junk imitation when the genuine article is far cheaper and so readily available? If you have a garden it's actually free!

The value of fruit is recorded in folklore: 'An apple a day keeps the doctor away.' When I was a boy a comment you often heard was: 'They were so rich, they had fruit in the house even when no-one was ill.'

CONSIDER THE IMPLICATIONS

Fruit has so much to recommend it in terms of taste, vitamins, nutrients, fibre, liquidity, absorption of energy, ease of digestion and disposal of toxins. Fresh fruit, supplemented with nuts, vegetables, grain and certain other vegetation, is clearly the food package Mother Nature designed for us.

After all, if we were supposed to eat junk foods such as meat, surely those would be the foods that would taste the best. If you still *do* believe they taste the best, how do you explain our need for condiments such as mustard and horseradish? Why do we have to smother junk food in ketchup or brown sauce? Why the need for salt and pepper? Why do we feel the need to spice up junk foods with strong flavours such as curry or garlic? If you eat food that's flavoured with garlic, you can't taste the food, just the garlic.

NATURAL IS BEST

We put additives in food either to disguise a foul taste or jazz up a bland taste.

Natural foods need no additives. They taste great in their entirely natural state with nothing added and nothing taken away.

THE FINAL PROOF

No food types have a higher liquid, energy and nutrient content than fruit. The high-liquid content facilitates rapid digestion, absorption of nutrients and disposal of wastes, resulting in maximum energy gain. That's why, when they want a quick burst of energy, tennis players eat bananas, and footballers eat oranges. Although fruits are technically solids they consist mainly of water. The high water-content supplies precious oxygen to the body. And have you noticed that even on the hottest of days, fresh fruit is not only refreshing but cool? Manufactured drinks will only be cool if they've been refrigerated or contain ice.

'WHAT ABOUT STRAWBERRIES AND CREAM?'

It's all part of the hype. Cream has a very bland taste and is seldom eaten on its own. Sugar is commonly sprinkled on strawberries and added to other fruit when unripe, thus converting it to junk. Only eat fruit when it's fresh and ripe. Avoid canned fruit immersed in sweetened syrup.

When they hear what's in Mother Nature's food package, some people worry that they will be forced to become vegetarians, or be deprived of variety in their diet. So let me dispel these fears.

THIS FEAR OF LACK OF VARIETY IS UNFOUNDED

In fact, many people experience very little variety in their diet, and before I discovered Easyweigh I was no exception. Breakfast used to consist of a bowl of cereal. I would eat the same cereal day after day. Occasionally I'd get fed up with cornflakes and switch to Weetabix or Shredded Wheat – then I would eat those every day. It's the same whether you have porridge, a fry-up, or a continental breakfast – most people tend to eat the same thing day after day.

Even with other meals the variation is not nearly as wide as we imagine. This dawned on me while browsing the menu at my favourite Indian restaurant. They were busier than usual and the waiter started to predict my selections. I asked how he knew what I wanted and he replied that the things he'd mentioned were what I always chose.

HEALTHY IS HAPPY

I realized then that in most of my favourite restaurants I would plough laboriously through the menu and end up ordering the same things each time!

There's nothing wrong with eating your favourite foods again and again, as long as they provide the energy and nutrients to keep you happy and healthy.

'WILL I BECOME A VEGETARIAN?'

Only if and when you want to. But let me reassure you that if you do choose to become vegetarian, there is a quite dizzying array of absolutely delightful flavours to select from. With the range of fruits, vegetables, nuts, seeds and vegetarian dishes now on offer in our supermarkets, you could dine for a month as a vegetarian without consuming the same dish twice. Many meat-eaters, by contrast, limit themselves to about four or five different types of meat: perhaps chicken, beef, lamb, pork, and turkey, with the occasional bit of seafood if they're feeling adventurous.

YOU WILL EXPERIENCE ALL THE VARIETY THAT YOU DO NOW, IF NOT MORE

Let me remind you of the junk margin: Easyweigh imposes no restrictions. I am not saying that you can only eat fruit, nuts and veg. I am saying that those foods are the ideal.

Either you already eat Mother Nature's foods, in which case you can enjoy the same variety that you do now – or you need to increase the percentage of these foods. On the other hand, if you're anything like I was before I discovered Easyweigh, you probably eat very little real food – in which case you will experience a far greater variety.

But there are certain kinds of junk food that you need to be a bit wary of.

REFINED FOODS

The process of refining food tends to remove most of the nutrients, vitamins and fibre. The worst culprits are highly refined carbohydrates: sugar, white rice and white flour. These foods make you fat because they supply only empty, low-quality calories, and excessive carbohydrates that are converted to fat.

BLOOD SUGAR BLUES

In the long run, highly refined carbohydrates create blood sugar *lows*, which we experience as lethargy, irritability and even depression. The 'lift' that people experience upon eating a sugary or starchy snack is an illusion – it's really just the momentary ending of the low brought about by the previous fix. It's like wearing tight shoes to enjoy the relief of taking them off.

If you wish to eat pasta, bread and rice, I suggest that where available you eat wholemeal bread and pasta, and wholegrain rice.

PHONEY FLAVOURS

Chocolate addicts tell me they adore the taste of chocolate, and in the same breath beg me to help them stop eating it, because they know it's making them fat and miserable! That just doesn't add up: even if chocolate were the most delightful taste in the world, that wouldn't explain why people keep eating it when it's clearly ruining their lives. No single taste can be worth your health and happiness.

Chocolate is a combination of three junk foods: cocoa, refined sugar to disguise the bitter taste, and milk, if it's milk chocolate. Cocoa contains a drug called theobromine, which combined with the addictive effect of the sugar compels you to go on eating it even after you've become sick of the taste.

Perhaps you think the addictive effect of chocolate is so great you can't resist it. But addictive substances can only affect you if you take them. No one's forcing you to eat it.

WOULD YOU EAT DEAD MICE?

Imagine scoffing half a box of chocolates then being told the centres consisted of dead mouse that had been minced and flavoured. Would you have any desire to consume the rest?

Theobromine is far worse for you than dead mouse.

WHERE DID IT ALL GO WRONG?

The brainwashing process began back in the mists of time, but it's got a lot worse in the last 200 years. For most of human history the majority of people have lived off the land in the countryside. But with the industrial revolution more and more people moved to the city. Back then fresh fruit and vegetables were not readily available in the city, and as a result we became more and more dependent on preserved junk. With the advent of TV advertising, the country dwellers became as brainwashed as everyone else.

The good news is that modern transport means that real food is easily available again for most of us. But people seem to have a basic need to interfere with nature: we are now modifying the genetics of natural food! That's like an ape attempting to fix a computer that isn't broken!

DON'T BELIEVE THE HYPE

The question is: are you going to continue to
fall for a con that will drastically reduce the
length and quality of your life?

'WHY DO SWEET THINGS TASTE GOOD?'

For the same reason that we like fruit: Mother Nature designed us that way. Ripe fruit tastes sweet, so she provided us with a sweet tooth to ensure we eat it. Is it her fault that people deceive themselves by adding fruit flavours and junk sweeteners to pass off junk food as the real thing?

Beware exotic desserts and pastries. Delicate junk food that has been artificially sweetened is even more dangerous than stodgy junk. In both cases your body lacks the essential nutrients and energy, and you still feel hungry. But because you don't feel bloated after eating light dishes, you're more likely to keep eating in a vain attempt to try and satisfy your hunger.

DON'T JUMP THE GUN

Do not proceed further unless you are certain that you both understand and agree with the principles I have outlined. Remember they are not mine. I make no claim to expert knowledge. I merely claim to have the common sense to understand and trust an evolutionary system that is a billion times more powerful than our own intelligence.

The third instruction is this: if you do not understand or agree with the principles I have outlined, re-read the book from the start.

THERE'S NO NEED TO RUSH IT!

You might understand the principles so clearly that you're tempted to switch to natural foods immediately. But any major change in life is followed by a little disorientation – even when it's a change for the better, like this one. Both your body and brain need time to adjust. The best approach is to proceed at a comfortable pace. That way you'll enjoy life right from the start.

'HOW DO YOU REMOVE THE BRAINWASHING?'

Use your common sense. No matter how eminent the authority, question everything you hear and read about food. If it contradicts the evolutionary system that designed us, as manifested in the principles outlined in this book, then ignore it. The process of reversing the brainwashing involves a two-pronged attack. Both prongs should be carried out simultaneously.

THE FIRST PRONG

Whenever you eat meat, fowl, fish or dairy products, remember the problems you create for your body. Consciously taste them without any additives. See those fancy desserts, pastries and sweets for the sickly concoctions of junk that they really are. You'll soon see the traditional breakfast of sausage, bacon and egg for what it really is: a plateful of indigestible grease!

THE SECOND PRONG

When you bite into a lovely, juicy piece of ripe fruit, savour the refreshing taste, and realize that it's packed with the energy and nutrients that you need to enjoy a long, healthy life. Relish the thirst-quenching properties of that vital high water content. Appreciate the fact that it's quickly and easily digested, and contains a minimum of waste.

IS EASYWEIGH PRACTICAL?

After all you can't hang about all day like a gorilla and eat a banana whenever you feel hungry! Fortunately you don't have to. Even wild animals have routines. Lions sleep all day and hunt in the evening. The trick is to establish a routine that satisfies your hunger and fits in with both your lifestyle and the principles of Easyweigh.

BE FLEXIBLE

The rest of the book will deal with the
practicalities of putting Easyweigh into effect.
Please don't think of these suggestions as
rigid rules that must be slavishly adhered to:
they are merely guidelines which, if followed
most of the time, will lead to permanent
weight loss and vibrant health.

GIVE YOUR DIGESTIVE SYSTEM A BREAK!

Although Mother Nature's food package contains a quite phenomenal range of flavours for you to enjoy throughout your life, it can be a mistake to consume too wide a variety of food types at any one time.

Pandas live exclusively on bamboo. Dogs, by contrast, will eat almost anything. We eat a variety of courses at one sitting, and each course – or indeed each mouthful – may well consist of a variety of different types of food, with added sauces and flavourings.

TIMING AND FRUIT

If fruit is eaten with foods other than fresh vegetables, it cannot be digested and putrefies in the stomach. This is one of the reasons some people have a bad reaction to certain fruits: it's because they have eaten it 'on top' of junk foods. When such people try eating fruit on an empty stomach, they usually find the adverse effects disappear.

Fruit may be included with simple green salads that contain no other ingredients such as meat, cheese, egg or tuna. Otherwise, try and make sure that you only eat fruit when your stomach is empty. Bear in mind that after a very heavy meal it can take up to eight hours for the stomach to empty.

FOOD COMBINING

Be wary of combining too many different types of food. If they are badly combined, eating too wide a variety of food types at the same meal causes serious problems in digestion, absorption of nutrients and disposal of waste.

The stomach uses acid-based juices to digest proteins, and alkaline-based juices to digest carbohydrates. Mix alkaline with acid and they neutralize each other. So, for example, if you eat a steak (protein) with a large portion of chips (carbohydrate), neither can be digested properly. The result is stagnation, indigestion and obesity.

KEEP YOUR BALANCE

This doesn't mean you have to separate proteins and carbohydrates completely. One of my favourite meals is wholemeal pasta (carbohydrate) with fresh pesto sauce and a few crushed nuts (protein) sprinkled on the top, with a salad on the side. That's fine. The idea is to avoid combining a *large* amount of protein with a *large* amount of carbohydrate at the same meal.

'HOW DO I GET STARTED?'

The best way is to eat fruit and only fruit for breakfast. Initially you might find the concept of a fruit breakfast difficult to accept, but this is because of the brainwashing. Be open-minded about it and in no time at all you'll wonder why you ever ate anything else.

If you eat three meals a day, a fruit breakfast means you've already achieved nearly half the 70 per cent natural food target.

'WILL I GET BORED WITH FRUIT?'

Termites don't get bored with rotting wood, and you'll only ever get bored with junk food. Experiment with the range of fruits on offer. Although the supermarkets have increased the range of junk, we can thank them for also introducing an incredible variety of delicious and exotic fruits and vegetables.

Just to give you some idea of the choice of fruits available to you there are apples, pears, cherries, oranges, tangerines, mangoes, bananas, grapefruits, strawberries, raspberries, blackberries, blackcurrants, redcurrants, gooseberries, lychees, melons, mulberries, kiwi fruits, grapes, pineapples, peaches, papayas, apricots and plums.

'WHAT ABOUT OTHER MEALS?'

Keep up the two-pronged attack to reverse
the brainwashing. Remember that we acquire
a taste for the foods that we eat regularly.
Set out deliberately to exploit that fact,
by experimenting with new flavours. Be
adventurous. Whether you're in a restaurant
or the supermarket, select fruits, vegetables
and dishes that you would previously have
dismissed. Remember that there's a junk
margin, so if you occasionally want a steak,
or some cheese or an omelette, that's OK.

'HOW DO I COMPUTE THE JUNK MARGIN?'

You don't have to. The simplest way to put Easyweigh into practice is to eat fruit for breakfast, and have a salad with every main meal. If you do that you can rest safe in the knowledge that roughly 70% of your intake is fresh, natural food. It doesn't matter if occasionally you exceed the 30% junk margin.

DON'T TURN THE SOLUTION INTO THE PROBLEM

If your job involves a lot of meals in hotels and restaurants, that needn't pose a problem. There are very few establishments that don't serve salad.

Easyweigh is flexible. Don't make a hassle of it. Remember: there are no rigid rules that must be followed all the time – merely guidelines to be followed most of the time. The appendix outlines the way to combine correctly. Try to do so where and when you can, but don't become a martyr to food combining, or indeed to any other aspect of Easyweigh.

My normal practice is to have fruit for breakfast, but away from home, I'll have something else if I can't get fruit. It's part of that all-important junk margin.

RECIPES

Easyweigh is a set of common sense principles, based on Mother Nature's good food guide, the application of which will enable you to achieve my claim. The method is designed to be flexible, in order to adapt to the lifestyle of each individual. It's neither my intention, nor within the scope of this book, to provide an extensive list of recipes. But I can offer a few suggestions.

SALADS

Here is just a small selection from the vast range of natural foods you might want to put in a salad: watercress, rocket, red onions, peppers, Chinese leaf, sun-dried tomatoes, baby sweet corn, artichoke hearts, pine nuts, sunflower seeds, cashew nuts, macadamias, pistachios, walnuts, olives, avocados, melon, orange, peach, grapes and pineapple.

It's OK to use a little bit of mayonnaise as part of your junk margin, but I far prefer healthier dressings such as olive oil and balsamic vinegar, lemon juice and olive oil, or fresh pesto.

JUST A COUPLE OF SUGGESTIONS

One of my favourite lunches is an avocado, lettuce and tomato sandwich, served on wholemeal bread with a smidgeon of pesto. Or I might have home-made guacamole (avocado, tomato, onion, chilli pepper, garlic and lemon juice, mixed in the blender) on wholemeal toast. For our evening meal my wife Joyce might stir fry some lovely fresh vegetables, or we might have baked potatoes with a crisp, fresh salad. If you sometimes want a steak or chicken breast or piece of fish with salad, that's OK. Alternatively salad can be the main feature of a meal, perhaps served in warmed wholemeal pitta bread, or wrapped in a tortilla. If you feel you need further inspiration, get a good salad recipe book. I find great pleasure in experimenting and discovering new recipes.

'I'M THE COOK IN THE HOUSEHOLD AND I CAN'T FORCE MY FAMILY TO EAT NATURAL FOODS'

It would be a mistake to even try to. But you do have a duty to try and convert them, and they'll thank you for it when they receive the benefits. Use some guile to change their eating habits gradually and they'll hardly even be aware that you're doing so.

NATURAL TASTES BEST

Remember that underneath all the brainwashing natural foods taste the best, so use a bit of ingenuity in conjuring up healthy meals that look and taste great, and they'll soon learn to love those foods.

'SHOULD I AVOID THE CHRISTMAS DINNER?'

Not if you don't want to. There's no harm in the occasional blow-out. But once you've learned to satisfy your hunger with real food, you'll find that stuffing yourself with vast amounts of junk no longer holds any appeal. I eat the same Christmas meal as the rest of the family, but I have a salad with it, and I eat slowly, savouring the taste of the food, and stop when I feel satisfied.

DON'T SNACK BETWEEN MEALS

It's usually done out of habit or boredom
and will ruin your precious hunger.
Overeating is not a cure for boredom. On
the contrary it leads to obesity and lethargy,
which reduces activity and therefore causes
boredom. A fit and healthy mind and body
should never be bored.

If you find yourself hungry between meals,
it's for one of two reasons. Either you're
not getting enough nutrients at those meals,
in which case you know the solution. The
other possible explanation is that you really
are going too long without eating. If your
lifestyle dictates that you have to go a long
time between meals, it's perfectly all right to
eat fruit between meals.

BEVERAGES

You might want to invest in a juicer. Some people prefer to juice their fruit in the morning, which is fine, but don't overdo it: just drink enough to quench your thirst and satisfy your hunger. A juicer can also come in handy for making vegetable juice, which can be drunk at mealtimes.

But by far the best thirst-quencher is cool, clear, cleansing, refreshing, oxygen-packed water. It's better to drink mineral water, but tap water is less harmful than a lot of things you could be drinking.

If you want the odd glass of wine with your meal, or an occasional cup of tea or coffee, that's OK as part of your junk margin – but don't kid yourself that any of these things will quench your thirst, because they won't.

MOTHER NATURE'S GUIDE TO DRINK

Drink when you're thirsty, and quench that thirst with water, or failing that with fruit or vegetable juices.

If you're not dehydrated, you rarely need to drink more than one glass of water at a time. Six would make you sick. Yet heavy drinkers can down eight pints of beer and still be thirsty.* That's because alcohol is diuretic, which means it dehydrates you. Tea, coffee and other caffeinated drinks such as colas have exactly the same effect. If any of these things appears to quench your thirst it's because the main ingredient is water! In the long run the diuretic effect will make you even thirstier.

*If you're worried about your alcohol consumption, I suggest you read one of my books on alcohol, or attend an Easyway clinic, details of which you'll find at www.allencarr.com.

COFFEE AND TEA

Some people drink 16 cups of tea or coffee a day, chiefly because of caffeine addiction. The main symptoms of caffeine withdrawal are lethargy and concentration problems. The 'boost' you get from a cup of tea or coffee is merely the temporary suppression of the caffeine withdrawal from the previous cup. Did I mention something earlier about wearing tight shoes to get a boost when you take them off?

If you want real energy, have a banana!

REVERSE THE BRAINWASHING

The world's healthiest, most refreshing drink isn't good enough for humans. We have to add colour, sugar, alcohol, caffeine and other junk. We crown it with a little umbrella and have the gall to feel superior to other species!

The process for reversing the brainwashing requires the same two-pronged attack as for food. When you drink tea, coffee, cola or alcoholic drinks, notice that they only appear to quench your thirst. That's why you have to drink so much of them, and it's why you feel thirsty again shortly afterwards. By contrast, notice that when you're genuinely thirsty the one thing that really hits the spot is cool, clear, refreshing, life-giving water.

USEFUL TIPS

Don't put too much food on your plate.
Ask yourself how hungry you really are. You
can always come back for more later – the
food's not going to run away! Take time to
savour your food, and when you have eaten
a plateful, just enjoy a few moments' peace
and quiet before you ask yourself whether
you're still hungry and need to eat more.

If someone serves you too much food, don't
attempt to clear your plate just because it's
there. Ask yourself: 'Do I really need to eat
more?' If the answer is 'No', stop eating.
You'll feel better for it and enjoy the next
meal far more.

EXERCISE

Most experts claim that exercise is essential
for weight reduction. Try telling that to a
tortoise. To exercise purely to lose weight
is part of the diet syndrome. It becomes
a penance and requires willpower. It's like
driving your car just to burn fuel. There's a
serious flaw in the idea that exercise can be
used as a direct means to the end of weight
loss. Your car with a full tank will weigh a
certain amount. If you drive the car and burn
all the fuel, the overall weight of the vehicle
will be less. But if you want to drive the car
again, you've got to re-fuel. In other words
exercise burns energy and dehydrates you:
this makes you hungry and thirsty, which
causes you to eat and drink more.

DRIVE YOUR CAR BECAUSE IT'S FUN TO DRIVE

I strongly recommend exercise, not to lose weight but because it will tone up your muscles, make you fit and healthy, and help you to enjoy life more. I shouldn't waste money on an exercise bike, rowing machine, or any other gimmicks. That would be part of the 'driving your car to burn fuel' syndrome – with the added absurdity that the vehicle doesn't actually go anywhere! It's much better to take up a sport, pastime or hobby that you enjoy. These days there's a huge variety of activities to choose from. Again, be adventurous. Try something you would previously have dismissed.

STAY FIT AND ACTIVE

Some of the things I have enjoyed in my
time are golf, tennis, squash, badminton,
walking, running, dancing, rowing, swimming
and table tennis. Most of these activities can
become an extremely enjoyable part of your
social life. But a word of warning: if you're
currently very unfit, consult your doctor
first, and build up your fitness level gently
and gradually. Since I became a Spanish
National Champion at the ripe old age of 68,
I think bowls should be included in my list of
activities.

IT'S YOUR CHOICE

A human being is a magnificent thing.
The human brain and body are capable
of astonishing feats, and the power of the
human spirit is virtually limitless.

We have all been given the precious gift of
human life, and it's up to each of us to decide
what we do with it.

I believe that every one of us has the
potential to live an extremely successful,
fulfilling life. That doesn't mean to say that
we all have to become jet-setting hot-shots.
There are different definitions of success.

The trick is to find out what you really want,
and – providing you don't hurt other people
along the way – use the very considerable
resources at your disposal to get it.

NEW LEVEL OF ENERGY

But you can't build a house on a swamp. If you continue to eat in a way that doesn't give you the energy and nutrients you need, you will be severely limiting those resources. On the other hand, if you put the principles outlined in this book into practice, in a very short time you will discover a level of energy that will astound you.

**THE REWARDS ARE ENORMOUS –
ENJOY LIFE!**

THE PRINCIPLES FOR CORRECT COMBINING

Avoid eating fruit with any food other than fresh vegetables.

Avoid combining a large amount of carbohydrates with a large amount of protein at the same meal. Carbohydrates are such things as starchy vegetables (potatoes, yams and sweetcorn etc.) and grains and grain products (wheat, rice, bread, pasta etc). Meat, poultry, fish, dairy products, eggs and nuts are all proteins.

KEEP IT SIMPLE

Avoid eating too many different types of
food and no more than one type of junk
food at any one meal.

Salads and other non-starchy vegetables can
be digested by either acid or alkaline juices
so they can be mixed with either proteins or
carbohydrates.

TELL ALLEN CARR'S EASYWAY
ORGANISATION THAT YOU'VE ESCAPED
Leave a comment on www.allencarr.com, email
yippee@allencarr.com, like our Facebook page
www.facebook.com/AllenCarr
or write to the Worldwide Head Office address
shown below.

ALLEN CARR'S EASYWAY CLINICS
The following list indicates the countries where
Allen Carr's Easyway To Stop Smoking Clinics
are currently operational. Check www.
allencarr.com for latest additions to this list.
The success rate at the clinics, based on the
three month money-back guarantee, is over 90
per cent.

Selected clinics also offer sessions that deal
with alcohol, other drugs, and weight issues.
Please check with your nearest clinic, listed
below, for details.

Allen Carr's Easyway guarantees that you will
find it easy to stop at the clinics or your money
back.

ALLEN CARR'S EASYWAY
Worldwide Head Office
Park House, 14 Pepys Road, Raynes Park,
London SW20 8NH ENGLAND
Tel: +44 (0)208 9447761
Email: mail@allencarr.com
Website: www.allencarr.com

Worldwide Press Office
Tel: +44 (0)7970 88 44 52
Email: media@allencarr.com

UK Clinic Information and Central Booking
Line 0800 389 2115 (Freephone)

UNITED KINGDOM	LEBANON
REPUBLIC OF IRELAND	LITHUANIA
AUSTRALIA	MAURITIUS
AUSTRIA	MEXICO
BELGIUM	NETHERLANDS
BRAZIL	NEW ZEALAND
BULGARIA	NORWAY
CANADA	PERU
CHILE	POLAND
COLOMBIA	PORTUGAL
CZECH REPUBLIC	ROMANIA
DENMARK	RUSSIA
ESTONIA	SERBIA
FINLAND	SINGAPORE
FRANCE	SLOVAKIA
GERMANY	SLOVENIA
GREECE	SOUTH AFRICA
GUATEMALA	SOUTH KOREA
HONG KONG	SPAIN
HUNGARY	SWEDEN
ICELAND	SWITZERLAND
INDIA	TURKEY
IRAN	UAE
ISRAEL	UKRAINE
ITALY	USA
JAPAN	

Visit www.allencarr.com to access your
nearest clinic's contact details.

OTHER ALLEN CARR PUBLICATIONS
Allen Carr's revolutionary Easyway method is
available in a wide variety of formats, including
digitally as audiobooks and ebooks, and has been
successfully applied to a broad range of subjects.

For more information about Easyway publications,
please visit
www.easywaypublishing.com

Lose Weight Now (with hypnotherapy CD)
ISBN: 978-1-84837-720-2

The Easy Weigh to Lose Weight
ISBN: 978-0-14026-358-9

Good Sugar Bad Sugar
ISBN: 978-1-78599-213-1

Stop Smoking Now (with hypnotherapy CD)
ISBN: 978-1-84837-373-0

Stop Smoking with Allen Carr (with 70-minute audio CD)
ISBN: 978-1-84858-997-1

The Illustrated Easy Way to Stop Smoking
ISBN: 978-1-84837-930-5

Finally Free!
ISBN: 978-1-84858-979-7

The Easy Way for Women to Stop Smoking
ISBN: 978-1-84837-464-5

The Illustrated Easy Way for Women to Stop Smoking
ISBN: 978-1-78212-495-5

How to Be a Happy Non-Smoker
ISBN: 978-0-572-03163-3

No More Ashtrays
ISBN: 978-1-84858-083-1

Smoking Sucks (Parent Guide with 16 page pull-out comic)
ISBN: 978-0-572-03320-0

The Little Book of Quitting
ISBN: 978-1-45490-242-3

The Only Way to Stop Smoking Permanently
ISBN: 978-0-14-024475-1

The Easy Way to Stop Smoking
ISBN: 978-0-71819-455-0

How to Stop Your Child Smoking
ISBN: 978-0-14027-836-1

The Easy Way to Control Alcohol
ISBN: 978-1-84837-465-2

No More Hangovers
ISBN: 978-1-84837-555-0

No More Fear of Flying
ISBN: 978-1-78404-279-0

The Easy Way to Stop Gambling
ISBN: 978-1-78212-448-1

No More Gambling
Ebook

No More Worrying
ISBN: 978-1-84837-826-1

Allen Carr's Get Out of Debt Now
ISBN: 978-1-84837-98-7

No More Debt
Ebook

The Easy Way to Enjoy Flying
ISBN: 978-0-71819-458-3

Burning Ambition
ISBN: 978-0-14103-030-2

Packing It In The Easy Way (the autobiography)
ISBN: 978-0-14101-517-0

DISCOUNT VOUCHER FOR
ALLEN CARR'S EASYWAY CLINICS

Recover the price of this book when
you attend an
Allen Carr's Easyway Clinic
anywhere in the world.

Allen Carr has a global network
of clinics where he guarantees
you will find it easy to stop
smoking or your money back.

The success rate based on this
money-back guarantee is over 90 per cent.

When you book your appointment
mention this voucher and you will
receive a discount to the value
of this book. Contact your
nearest clinic for more information
on how the sessions work and
to book your appointment.
Not valid in conjunction with any other offer.